Your Free Gift!

I want to say thank you for buying my book so I put together a free gift for you!

This gift is a perfect compliment for the book, it's a little bonus recipe you can use around your house!

Just Visit The Link Below And Download It Totally Free!

http://lucrativelifepublishing.com/free-gift-pure-health/

I hope you enjoy this awesome treat.

Thank You For Supporting My Work.

Sydney Summers

Table of Contents

Western versus Natural Medicine

If you go far enough back in time, there was only "natural medicine". Before mankind knew in detail the intricacies of his own anatomy or the mechanics of viruses and bacteria in the body, he relied on folk wisdom and the botanical knowledge handed down by lay people.

The trial and error of figuring out that a plant had therapeutic value was a long and arduous process. Physiological health was something closely wrapped up in superstition, religious beliefs and was understood to be up to the whimsy of the gods.

In time, however, people learnt to study the natural world around them in greater detail, and learnt to isolate exactly what compounds were useful in things like willow bark or calendula flowers. Very gradually, what was once a subtle art form practiced at home or by healers who passed their wisdom down to apprentices became a science – a science that could be monetized, optimized and trademarked.

The important thing about "Western" medicine is that there is no such thing – evidence based treatments that rely on peer-reviewed studies and hard experimental proof have no cultural element – it is merely medicine.

So why is there an enormous rift between ancient, holistic wisdom handed down from generations and the more legitimate arena of "Western medicine"? While evidence based medicine, the kind you will receive if you consult a GP today, is the best that mankind has to offer when it comes to our health, it is not always the full story.

Western medicine grew from the ancient knowledge of natural therapeutic treatments, and to this day continues to be inspired by several of its key principles. While antibiotics, for example, were hailed as a medical science triumph in the early 40s, today we know what many natural healers have understood for thousands of years – that the body is in fact a highly complex system and that it is not possible to merely swoop in, destroy one particular microorganism and then swoop out without disturbing the ecology of the entire human GI tract.

You will not find in this book any critique of Western medicine, as its methods have saved more lives than any other healing paradigm. At the same time, "natural" medicine (that is, the kind of healing practices that don't readily fit into a capitalistic, pathology focused and synthetic mode of treatment) usually shines where Western medicine fails.

Here, we will consider gentler, more organic (in the sense that they originate from plant materials) and supportive treatments – the kind that fall under the preventative umbrella and take into consideration the fact the human body is not simply a machine.

While a conventional doctor cannot consult with you for a mere 20 minutes and determine that you require a different diet, more exercise and more meaningful connections with your family, *you* can take this aspect of your health into your own hands. By becoming curious about the value of the plants and natural ingredients around us, we can simultaneously tune our ear to the messages our body's are sending us, and find ways to nurture and support our own innate health and vitality.

Advantages of Natural Medicine

Botanical extracts and supplements are no substitute for proper medical care, especially when it comes to injuries. However, the methods we'll discuss below greatly increase your body's chances of resisting and recovering from illness in the first place. In fact, the treatments outlined below encompass so great an area that they are more akin to a lifestyle than a brief intervention that you stop after your symptoms disappear.

Natural medicine is:

- Holistic. Your "mental health" is not a separate category from the rest of you, for example. It is not absurd to acknowledge that your social anxiety, irritable bowel and occasional acne flare-ups are all related – and to choose a treatment that doesn't address each individual symptom but the underlying source of *all* the symptoms.
- Cumulative. You don't take a course of natural medicine quite like you do with antibiotics; rather, you craft your health and well being constantly, over the long term.
- Free – in the sense that you require no special licenses or degrees to access and make use of the information. Of course, this also means that you need to do your homework and take mature responsibility for what you put into your body.
- Variable. When you are dealing with synthetic medications, you are dealing with a pre-made, distilled, usually synthetic and isolated compound. Plants, on the other hand, differ greatly depending on the soil they grew in, their harvesting method, species and what other plants they are combined with. The complexity of herbal treatments means we need to approach them with respect and caution.
- Not all that different from a healthy diet in general. For the holistic natural healer, food is medicine and medicine is food. Everything that can be consumed either supports or undermines the integrity of the body, and so all foods have the potential to have therapeutic effects on the body.

The rest of this book will focus largely on herbal and botanical ingredients as these are the most numerous and easiest to use.

Where to Buy Herbs and How to Store Them

To store dried and preserved herbs

For the vast majority of therapeutic botanicals, the active compounds can be found in the oils, fats or fatty acids in the plant. Different plants respond differently to being dried, boiled, steamed or pressed, so it's important to know exactly how to store and contain preserved herbs so that their natural essences are preserved. Store herbs out of direct sunlight and away from moisture, steam etc. Glass jars kept in the pantry are always a good bet.

Mountainroseherbs.com has a large and devoted following; also check out herbaffair.com.

To store your own fresh herbs

If you've grown herbs yourself, they are quite simple to dry. Here are a few methods:

- Chop the plant up finely and then spread in a single layer onto a baking tray and put into the oven at the lowest possible heat for a few hours. Check on them periodically to make sure they are not scorching. Do not wash herbs first as the moisture will interfere with the drying process and may even introduce mold. When you're done, crumble gentle and store in a dark glass far away from sunlight and moisture. Herbs stored this way will keep for about 6 months, losing their flavor and essence after that.
- For oily herbs like lavender or rosemary, simply string them up and hang in a dry and airy cupboard, away from light. Leave as is or crumble into a jar as above. Make sure that they are not covered in dust before you use them!

For all herbs, always remove yellow or brown leaves and make sure they are clean and have no tiny insects hiding in the leaves. Be vigilant for any signs of mold on dried herbs and throw out if you detect a strange smell. It also pays to label things clearly especially if you don't trust your memory/nose to help you identify a herb later on.

The Treasure Chest of Herbs

So, let's dive in!

The information out there about herbs and their uses is vast and would take many lifetimes to learn and understand fully. Nevertheless, there are a few tried and true herbal remedies that are relatively safe and highly effective, even for beginners.

Below is a list of the most popular and readily available herbs that anyone can begin to use to improve their health and wellness without relying on harsh and synthetic medications. Naturally, you can use these herbs in blends and with methods of your own design after you feel comfortable working with them and are more confident in how they interact with your own unique constitution.

Before we begin, a broad warning: most of the herbs on the following list are not advisable for use with pregnant or breastfeeding women. If you're experiencing any heart, liver or kidney complications, the onus is on you to research carefully how a particular plant will interact with both your condition and any medications you may be taking for it. Remember that just because something is natural, it doesn't mean it can't hurt you.

The Calming and Mood Altering Plants

The following herbs are excellent for soothing nervous tension, anxiety, stress, worry, insomnia, shock and symptoms of PMS.

Chamomile

German chamomile is the most popular. Brew a tablespoon in hot water for a soothing tea to calm insomnia or depression. The flower heads are the best part of the plant to use, although the leaves are active, too.

Catnip

Another excellent sedative – and not just for cats! Make a tea or tincture for a calming remedy that promotes a mild sense of euphoria.

Lavender

Probably the most versatile herb in the world. Lavender has remarkable effects on mood and can be used in any blend intended to balance, refresh and anchor. Used in teas, oils, all beauty preparations and cleaning products, there's nothing lavender can't do. Place a drop on your pillow to help you sleep.

St. John's Wort

Plenty of peer-reviewed studies confirm St. John's Wort's place as a viable remedy for anxiety and depression. Excellent for PMS and general tension and great used either as a tea or in capsule form – although be careful as it does interfere with other medications, the contraceptive pill included. Be patient; St. John's Wort does take some time to build up in the system.

Oat Straw

Used also as an aphrodisiac as it boosts free testosterone in the blood, oat straw lifts the spirits and is a good treatment for stress and anxiety. Brew a tablespoon as a daily tea. Rich in vitamins and minerals, a morning cup of oat straw tea is good for mild anxiety.

Borage

Delicious and energising, and popular in Mediterranean cusine. A good daily treatment for depression.

Energising Plants

Citrus – lemon, grapefruit, bergamot

All citrus is used in aromatherapy to brighten, lift moods, cleanse, tone, refresh and stimulate. Bergamot is famous for flavouring Earl Grey Tea. Lemon and grapefruit are useful for degreasing and cleansing, and orange blossom is used in all perfumes and massage blends to soften and brighten.

Dot some oil onto your wrists when your energy is flagging, or burn with a carrier oil in a ceramic burner when you need to focus and work. On waking every morning, a glass of spring water with the juice of one lemon or grapefruit will wake you up and leave you feeling fresh and ready to tackle the day.

Pine

A clear, strong and unisex ingredient in any aromatherapy treatment, pine is a good addition to cleaning preparations and energising diffusor blends.

Pine needles can also be made into an antibiotic tea. To make a very effective tincture for a cough or sore throat, take 1 tablespoon of fresh pine needles, chop and smash into smaller pieces and then boil in water about 20 minutes to make a strong tea, and drink.

The same tea, when cooled, can be used as a poultice to encourage healing on bruised, burnt, and inflamed skin. Pine oil, when massaged into the skin with another milder carrier oil, can relieve bronchitis, pneumonia, bronchitis and rheumatic pain – just be careful not to get any into broken skin.

Making your own pine oil is easy: simply submerge pine needles in olive oil and simmer on low heat for around 25 minutes. This oil is healing but also very refreshing to have in the home as part of your home made cleaning recipes. Add a few drops of pine oil and lemon

oil to water to wash down surfaces and leave them smelling lovely –
without using any chemical-laden detergents.

Rosemary

Refreshing and stimulating, a little rosemary goes a long way. Good
for hair rinses, plenty of roasting recipes, aromatherapy blends and
a good oil to diffuse.

Antibiotic and Immune Strengthening Ingredients

Echinacea

A popular herb known to have been used by ancient American Indians for chest complications, colds, flus, coughs and to strengthen the immune system. Interestingly, Echinacea is a robust grower and can be easily cultivated at home.

Nettle

Incredibly nutritious and full of vitamins and minerals, nettle tea also helps with acne and hormone conditions. Also supports the immune system.

Honey

Antiseptic, antibacterial, antiviral and antifungal. Honey, when combined with a little water, creates a small amount of hydrogen peroxide, which can lighten and sterilize. For cuts or grazes, a thin layer of honey spread over will prevent infection, keep out dirt and particles and speed healing.

Garlic

Excellent for colds and flus, and belongs in everyone's diet. Raw garlic is best. Combine with parsley if the garlic-breath is an issue.

Ginger

Along with its cousin galangal, ginger is incredibly rich in antioxidants. A simple tea of fresh ginger in water will quell nausea, but add honey and lemon if treating a cold or sore throat.

Goldenseal

An expensive and rather difficult herb to get hold of, goldenseal is nevertheless an excellent general antibiotic, antiviral and antimicrobial. Use in small quantities as a tea or tincture to treat acute viral infections.

Clove

A good antimicrobial. Can be used effectively to numb a toothache: Take a few whole cloves and put in the mouth close to the painful tooth and wait a while for your saliva to soften it. After a while, chew on the cloves slowly to release their healing oil, focusing on the sore tooth. It should go numb after a while – and prevent infection from spreading.

Antioxidant Plants

Turmeric

Another cousin of the miraculous ginger. Add turmeric to tea, soups or Indian/Asian dishes for an intense shot of plant phenols. Make a strong tea of turmeric and crushed fresh fenugreek seeds for upset stomachs, or make a paste with olive oil to create a hair mask that helps soothe dandruff.

Blueberries

Blueberries are still use din parts of the world for their power to calm stomach troubles. They're also very nutritious and rich in fiber and antioxidants. Add a few to your morning smoothie.

Rosehips

By weight, rosehips have the highest vitamin C content of any food. Make a syrup of fresh rose hips by boiling in water until all the juice is extracted. This is delicious in tea, or can be made into a jam by adding sugar. A decoction of rose hips combined with rose water and witch hazel makes a beautiful and gorgeous smelling skin toner.

Borage seed essential oil

Can be used in a carrier oil (jojoba, grape seed, coconut etc.) to treat eczema, dermatitis and swelling. Effective when combined with camphor or aloe. A few drops of the seed oil and a small amount of olive oil rubbed into the belly can soothe menstrual cramping.

A similar massage oil helps with rheumatoid arthritis. For a persistent cough, brew a strong tea of dried borage and drink very hot with a little honey. Combine with dried sage (an excellent expectorant and mucous clearer) for a tea that will soothe a ragged throat.

Hormone Balancing Plants

Red clover: rich in isoflavines that behave like estrogen in the body
Nettle: Relieves PMS, cramps and bloating, encourages milk
production and reduces bleeding
Sarsaparilla: Boosts the llibido and helps with urinary tract
infections
Ladies mantle: Soothes cramps and diarrhea
Chasteberry/vitex: Regulates hormone imbalances

A tea made of any or all of the above can be sipped throughout the
day around the time of your cycle to support your body's balance.

Digestive aids

Fennel

An excellent stomachic and carminative. Can be chewed after meals to freshen the breath and aid digestion, or else brewed into a tea, alone or with peppermint.

Peppermint

A good remedy for all symptoms of irritable bowel, bloating, gas and indigestion. A drop or two or peppermint oil in water taken before meals will promote good absorption.

Coconut oil

Coconut oil is a great way to get nutrition into the body when digestion is impaired for any reason. The medium chain fatty acids help to heal the digestive tract from the inside out; good for ulcers, bloating and leaky gut.

Plants That Heal The Skin

Marigold

Make a strong decoction of marigold/calendula flowers and bath wounds, bruises or grazes with it – marigold will soothe inflammation and speed healing, as well as keep the area clean and deter infection.

Camphor

Made from the camphor laurel tree, this waxy substance can be made synthetically (from mineral turpentine) but is best natural and organic. It has been used for centuries as a medicine, embalming fluid and even religious ritual scent.

While camphor is not safe to take orally, it is a great topical treatment to soothe pain and itching, or to treat fungal infections like cold sores, warts, and even haemorrhoids or mild burns. By increasing blood flow to an area, camphor acts to reduce irritation and swelling. Be careful not to apply to broken skin. Simply apply to affected areas and gently massage in.

Coconut oil

Coconut oil is the single substance on earth with the richest concentration of Lauric acid. Lauric acid breaks down in the human body into monolaurin, a healing and soothing fatty acid, the only other source of which is human breast milk. The medium chain fatty acids in coconut milk make it an excellent food for those weak or convalescing, and is a gold standard for treating Candida Albicans overgrowth.

If you suffer frequent bouts of thrush, poor digestion, skin trouble, lethargy and weight gain, you might have an overabundance of candida. A common but surprisingly effective regime to rebalance your internal gut flora is to eat coconut oil everyday.

Start with a few teaspoons and work your way up to as many as three tablespoons. Eat directly or add to cooking. Ensure that the oil is virgin, hydrogenated and unrefined – it should still smell like coconuts. In time, you'll experience bacterial "die off" as your body re establishes balance.

A daily shot of coconut oil is also excellent for encouraging weight loss as it boosts the metabolism and helps your body burn fat for energy instead of storing it. "Leaky gut syndrome", wherein food allergies or antibiotic overuse create tiny holes in the GI tract lining, is very effectively treated by coconut oil.

Be sure to also eat plenty of fermented foods (real sauerkraut, kimchi, kefir and yogurt are good choices) to repopulate your gut. It's no exaggeration to say that a healthy intestinal lining constitutes almost all of your body's immunity and can have consequences for your entire body.

Topically, coconut oil is a good treatment for osteoarthritis or any joint pain caused by infection of the joints. While traditional antibiotics cannot enter an infected joint since it is effectively sealed off from the bloodstream, coconut oil can be absorbed into the joint directly. There, the medium chain fatty acids literally break down the cell walls of harmful viruses, bacteria and microorganisms. To treat stiff and aching joints – even if it results from injury or over-exercise, massage a blend of coconut oil, camphor and any essential oil you like into the joint. This will lubricate the joint and go some way to restoring mobility.

Aloe

If you can get a hold of fresh aloe leaves, it can be incredibly healing to break open a leaf and smear the clear gel over fresh wounds, bites, scrapes, burns or even rashes. It will be slightly sticky. A prepared aloe gel is also an alternative and has a tightening, astringent effect on the skin, so is great for the oily T zone or to reduce shininess.

Plants Used For Cleaning

Apple cider vinegar

A good tip to keeping toilets super clean and shiny is to drop a cup of apple cider vinegar in the toilet bowl and allow it to stand over night. Scrub and flush in the morning for a clean toilet that smells faintly of apples.

Lemons

Cut a lemon in half. Sprinkle the raw edge with a mixture of coarse and fine salt. If you like, you can also add a sprinkle of bicarbonate of soda. Now, you have a makeshift lemon scrubber that degreases, disinfects and deodorizes bathtubs, tiles and other dirty surfaces, while leaving everything smelling very fresh. Drop a single drop of pine oil on top for an even lovelier scent.

Olive oil

For oil stains or stains from greasy food, make a paste with baking soda and olive oil to gently massage into the area. The oil will dissolve the oil in the stain and the baking soda acts as a mild detergent. Now, wash as normal and the stain will dissolve far quicker.

Soap nuts

Soap nuts contain their own natural saponin and can be added to loads of laundry as an alternative to washing detergent. After a few uses, their natural soap is depleted and then you can recycle the husks. Soap nuts are eco-friendly, scentless and very mild – and yes, they do work. Look online for a good online retailer – soap nut powder is also available.

Check out Amazon or organicsoapnuts.net

Plants Used For Beauty

For hair

Make a hair rinse with either chamomile tea (to lighten blonde hair) or rosemary oil (to add shine to darker hair) along with a cup of apple cider vinegar and a cup of brewed nettle tea. Don't rinse with water afterwards – the vinegar smell will dissipate as hair dries.

Color hair in shades of red by using henna powder. For a simple recipe, mix 100% pure and authentic henna powder with a little yogurt and lemon juice to make a past. Let it sit for a few minutes to develop and then apply as a hair mask to the hair.

Cover with cling wrap for an intensified color and rinse off after anything from 30 minutes to overnight depending on the desired color. A strand test is essential. Other things to add to the mix to alter the color: hibiscus petals, ground coffee, beet juice or honey.

To make a treatment for head live, buy a whole jar of coconut oil. Patiently comb the entire contents through the hair, making sure the scalp is covered well, too. Now, cover in a thick layer of cling wrap. The heat and lack of oxygen will help coconut oil to do its work. When you rinse it out, you'll also rinse away the lice. Add a few drops of tea tree oil if you have it.

For skin

For oily or acne prone skin, an astringent made of pure (not diluted) Witch hazel will control shine and sebum production. Dab a tiny drop of tea tree oil on pimples to dry them out quickly.

You can also make an effective face mask using a base of Rhassoul clay. To this add mashed papaya (the enzymes serve to remove the dead skin cells), a bit of honey to disinfect and prevent pustules for becoming infected, and a drop of calming lavender oil. Let this mask sit on the face for up to 30 minutes and rinse off.

A temporary tightening effect can be achieved under the eyes by painting on a small amount of egg white. Aloe Ferox gel (not vera, which is less potent, but Ferox, which is yellowish in color) can also be an effective remedy for wrinkles.

Freckles and sunspots can be gradually lightened with a mixture of lemon and honey. Be very careful as excessive use of lemon on the skin can lead to heightened photosensitivity, which ironically leads to more sunspots and freckles! Use a mix of equal parts honey and lemon, wipe lightly over the face, leave for no more than 2 minutes, then wash off thoroughly and moisturize.

Make your own lip tinted balm by combining a teaspoon of melted beeswax with a teaspoon of Shea butter and a few drops of hibiscus tincture or beet juice. This will give you a pretty, rosy color that actually seems to suit every skin type.

For very dry skin, melt a tablespoon of coconut oil and them combine with a half a mashed avocado. Leave on the skin for 10 or more minutes, then gently wash off. Moisturizer will usually not be necessary.

To treat sunburn, run a coolish bath with camphor leaves and a half-cup of apple cider vinegar in it. These two will help soothe burnt skin. Soak for a while without scrubbing. When you get out, rub over the affected skin with a cooled Ceylon tea bag. Pat yourself dry slightly and then smear over a liberal amount of both coconut oil and aloe vera gel.

For a really gorgeous shower time treat that leaves your skin glowing and soft, combine a half-cup of brown sugar with a teaspoon of cinnamon and then add either 1/3 cup melted coconut oil or extra virgin olive oil.

In the shower, use the scrub to slough off dead skin cells – the sugar and cinnamon will exfoliate and encourage blood flow while the oil moisturizes. You'll smell heavenly and be super soft after you dry yourself off. While you're in the shower, try rubbing a lemon half over elbows and knees – not only will the acid help to soften and remove dead skin cells, it'll also lighten any discoloration.

For teeth

Avoid putting acids like lemon on the teeth – though they will temporarily whiten the teeth, in time they corrode the enamel and will leave you with more stained teeth and sensitivity issues.

Instead, make a thin paste with bicarbonate of soda and gently brush the teeth with this, once a week until the desired results are reached. Alternatively, rub fresh strawberries over the teeth as often as you like for a subtle whitening effect.

For a simple but very effective breath freshener, chew on ½ teaspoon of fennel seeds along with a few sprigs of parsley – especially if you've just had a garlicky meal.

For nails

Soak the tips of nails in the juice of a freshly squeezed lemon for 5 minutes or so to white the tips. Scrub with a nailbrush. This treatment can be performed as often as you like. A drop of either coconut oil or jojoba oil rubbed into the cuticles will prevent hangnails and dry skin. Shea butter alone or combined with a few drops of essential oil makes a perfectly adequate hand cream.

A stronger nail whitening effect can be achieved with equal parts of 3% hydrogen peroxide and baking soda made into a paste. Apply to the whole nail and rinse off after a few minutes. This treatment can be performed every month or two as it's quite strong.

Why Organic?

The thing about botanical remedies is that they are nowhere near as standardized and regular as their synthetic counterparts. Just like a person, a plant will differ according to where it grows and how, as well as what specific species it is, whether it was sprayed with pesticides during its growth and the like.

A plant that has been grown in nutrient depleted soil, rushed through its growth cycle, doused with harmful pesticides etc. will not of course be as effective as a plant that is grown to its full potential in chemical free soil.

Wherever you can, buy organic. Be aware that some smaller companies may sell herbs that are actually organic but because of the size of the business, it doesn't make sense for them to pay to be certified by an organic certifying body. In this case, use your discretion and be curious about how the plants you consume are grown, harvested and stored.

Many manufacturers share your passion for properly grown organic produce and will be happy to chat about their process with you. Of course, another alternative is to grow what you can yourself. Get organic seeds and raise a few plants at home; in this way you can be absolutely sure of their quality.

The Importance of Nutrition

As mentioned earlier in this book, in real life, the line between medicinal herbs and those used for cooking blurs very quickly. Should you store coconut oil in the kitchen where you use it to cook with or in the bathroom where you use it as a facial moisturizer? Is ginger really to be considered a medicine when it is as delicious as it is and eaten often anyway?

As you move towards a more natural, unprocessed and holistic way of thinking about your own health and wellness, you'll unavoidably start to question your diet. Though each person will gravitate towards a way of eating that resonates most strongly with them and whatever works in their particular lifestyles, there are always fundamental principles of wellness that hold true for whatever your chosen diet is, be it Paleo, calorie controlled, vegan/vegetarian or whatever.

5 universal principles of a healthful regime of eating

- Honor your hunger. Support your body's own innate tendency towards wellness by listening closely to your appetite. Not your addictions and cravings, naturally, but to what truly serves your highest good. This means eating when you're hungry and not eating when you're full.
- Eat wholesome foods. There is no diet in the world that promotes the use of refined, over processed and synthetic foods. Whatever you eat, make sure it's the best quality you can manage.
- Vary your diet. Humans are omnivores. Whatever you decide to focus on, keep things interesting by getting a full range of as many different kinds of fresh plants as possible.
- Avoid toxins. A healthy diet means nothing if you're simultaneously binge drinking, smoking or regularly taking in heavy metals, pesticides or other additives.
- Stay hydrated. Water is basically your most primary and important foodstuff. Drink water liberally.

- Stay open minded. What works for you may not always work for others, and vice versa. Be happy to adjust and change as necessary.

Conclusion

Thank you again for downloading my book!

Hopefully in this short book you've been inspired by the health benefits of natural medicine and the organic remedies for a better and healither life. Living a healthy lifestyle doesn't have to be hard, nor does it have to be expensive! The best part about making your own home remedies is that its all super affordable and you aren't wasting any product!

If you are just starting out with natural medicine, try some of the simple remedies outlined here and gradually work your work up to more complicated measures, you will be amazed at the amount of medicine you can make. Nothing can beat the sense of satisfaction that comes with working *with* your body in natural and wholesome ways.

Finally, if you enjoyed this book, would you mind leaving me an honest review? Reviews are so important for authors like me and it would mean a huge amount to me if you took the 2 minutes to write one.

I do look forward in reading your review, thanks in advance.

Also, if you missed your Free Gift just flip to the next page to get it now!

Your Free Gift!

I want to say thank you for buying my book so I put together a free gift for you!

This gift is a perfect compliment for the book, it's a little bonus recipe you can use around your house!

Just Visit The Link Below And Download It Totally Free!

http://lucrativelifepublishing.com/free-gift-pure-health/

I hope you enjoy this awesome treat.

Thank You For Supporting My Work.

Sydney Summers

www.ingramcontent.com/pod-product-compliance
Lightning Source LLC
Chambersburg PA
CBHW060445290526
45793CB00002B/581